Eyesight Improvement

The 20/20

Vision Blueprint:

Improve Your Eyesight in 21 Days

Joanne Bateman

Disclaimer – Please Read!
The information provided in this book is designed to provide helpful information on the subjects discussed. This book is not meant to be used, nor should it be used, to diagnose or treat any medical condition. For diagnosis or treatment of any medical problems, consult your own physician. The publisher and author are not responsible for any specific health or allergy needs that may require medical supervision and are not liable for any damages or negative consequences from any treatment, action, application or preparation, to any person reading or following the information in this book. References are provided for informational purposes only and do not constitute endorsement of any websites or other sources. Readers should be aware that the websites listed in this book may change.

Eyesight Improvement: The 20/20 Vision Blueprint

CONTENTS

Eyesight Improvement: The 20/20 Vision Blueprint

CHAPTER 1 - EYENTRODUCTION

This book is not aimed at being the be-all and end-all for all things related to bad eyesight; rather, it's to be the best and most complete A-Z guide available on the market for improving your eyesight naturally. This book is geared towards those looking to improve their eyesight efficiently whilst keeping them in tip-top shape, without the aid of spectacles, contact lenses or expensive surgery – none of which are guaranteed methods of correcting our vision problems long-term. Bad eyesight has become so prevalent in today's society and we will look at why that is. A 2014 research study done by the National Eye Institute found that 75% of Americans use some form of corrective lens! 75% of people, that means more than 7 out of every 10 people you walk by uses some form of corrective lens, be it contacts or eye glasses.

The scary thing is that not everyone needs glasses and those who do need glasses often end up with a prescribed lens much stronger than what they require. Following *The 20/20 Vision Blueprint* presented in this book for just 21 days, you will notice an improvement in your vision, gain a more accurate prescription for your lenses and eventually avoid wearing prescription glasses for certain activities if you keep it up. *The 20/20 Vision Blueprint* has been structured to lessen the degree and frequency of any headaches you might currently be experiencing due to eyesight problems, reduce eye strain and improve your eyesight to its most optimal level naturally.

As most of you would know, once we get our first pair of correctional lenses, we go in for check-ups, be it every two years or in some instances yearly or less! The chances of someone being given correctional eye exercises, or being advised on lifestyle changes, are almost negligible, which is why this book is in your hands. With that being said however, if you have recently experienced failing eyesight or any severe eye traumas, you should make an appointment with your optometrist straight away. While *The 20/20 Vision Blueprint*, strategies and techniques outlined in this book will help you improve your eyesight it isn't the magic cure to all things related to bad eyesight.

You should consult a professional for any health related topics, including your eyes. This book is in no way meant to take the place of professional treatment.

We're confident you will find this book to be a valuable resource on your journey towards a better vision.

CHAPTER 2 - THE BIG ELEPHANT OPTOMETRISTS HAVE BEEN HIDING IN THE ROOM

Did you know the 'eyewear and eye care' industry in the US accounted for $15 billion in revenue in 2014? In the UK this figure drops to a more 'modest' £2.82 billion with Canada trailing close behind at $2.98 billion. Now you might be thinking that you know where this is headed but it's not the full picture!

I was a Store Manager at the local optometrists (hint: it starts with L and ends in A) for five years and in that time, there would be the rare customer who'd come in for their yearly checkup and score significantly better on their eye exam since their last checkup. These rare specimens would walk out with prescribed lenses much weaker then what they came in with. Needless to say this was a bit of a shock to me; after all doesn't eyesight just stay on level ground (if you're lucky!) or decline over time?

I brought this phenomenon up with several of the optometrists at the store when these customers had come in and the optometrists would always brush it off with the same lame excuses such as "We get this sometimes, some just get better at guessing the letters as time goes on" or "Yeah and?" as if it was no big deal. Needless to say, I wasn't overly impressed with these answers so I started talking to other colleagues and store managers that had been in the industry for a while. They all said similar things BUT one store manager mentioned something that piqued my interest, apparently he had a long chat with one of these phantom customers and they claimed to be doing eye exercises which improved their vision. I thought to myself eye exercises?

I wasn't waiting for the next miracle customer to walk in the store to tell me how they did it so I started digging around and decided to consult someone who I knew I could trust.

Dr. Google.

That's when I found out about the ophthalmologist William Bates, who wrote the book *Perfect Sight Without Glasses*. I raced through the book in a weekend and my mind was blown into smithereens, the book detailed a multitude of exercises to improve vision and included the causes of common eye problems along with their cures. There were a ton of other things covered in the book which we'll discuss in later chapters.

Come Monday, I was the most enthusiastic and pumped for work I had EVER been for a Monday. I couldn't wait to regurgitate and vomit this information all over everyone at work and see what they thought.

Talk about a turn of events, by lunch time I was in utter dismay; everyone I had spoken to either laughed or brushed off what I shared like it meant nothing. All everyone wanted to talk about was what they got up to on the weekend (including me!).

That's when John Newing (the editor of this book – thanks John!), a graduate optometrist at the time, joined me for lunch and brought up the topic. He had come across William Bates' work in college and had also brought his work to the attention of his lecturers. All of them reacted in the same manner that I faced at work. The more we got to talking about the exercises and credibility of them, the more I sensed that John was hiding something from me, he wanted to say something but wasn't sure if he should. I pestered him and gnawed at him till he finally spilled the beans and I couldn't believe it, I almost wished he hadn't told me.

In the morning team meeting between the optometrists they had brought up how I was 'prancing' around telling everyone about these eye exercises. Apart from being called some uncivil words, the real kicker was when they said they knew this stuff worked! Not only that but when customers had brought this topic up to them in the past, they would actually convince the customers that the exercises were all placebo. The chief optometrist then turned to John and said "You know people like Joanne wouldn't have her job if we didn't do this. Neither would you John, you wouldn't be able to pay off your student loans then could you?" He even had the audacity to throw a wink at John.

When I heard all of this I was absolutely outraged. Yes it's a known fact that some people act out of sheer profit but this was the first time it was smack bang right in my face, in person. People I knew were doing the complete opposite of what their job stood for, it didn't get any more raw then that.

This is why this book is now in your hands. Shortly after this debacle, I started secretly telling and explaining to customers the Bates Method and the different eye exercises they could do. I followed up with the majority of them a month or so after to see how they were doing; a few would even contact me beforehand telling me how this stuff actually worked. A vast amount of them (those that actually stuck to the exercises and tips!) reported that they noticed significant improvements and the majority actually ended up coming in for checkups earlier than scheduled so they could get weaker prescriptions as their old lenses weren't clear anymore! This book summarizes the exercises, instructions and guides I gave to customers and the subsequent groups of people that I taught. If *The 20/20 Vision Blueprint* is performed diligently, they will improve your vision naturally.

Please don't take my experience with optometrists the wrong way though! As with any demographic you have people who are the absolute scum of the Earth and there are also those who stand for and do what's right. This was clearly demonstrated by John and many other optometrists I have since connected with who actually encourage patients to try certain eye exercises or make lifestyle changes before settling on corrective eyewear. Not all optometrists are bad!

THE SPECTACLE WHEEL

So how does this whole industry operate and sustain itself?

Well, it all starts when people tend to start experiencing either blinding headaches or find that their vision starts getting blurry when they are reading things up close or far away such as road signs. And what's the first port of call for most people in these instances?

Damn, it's time for a visit to the optometrists, my eyes are getting worse it must be because of (insert excuse here – age, genes, watching too much TV, computer time etc). I have to get my eyes checked out and see how good (or bad) my vision actually is. Oh, look on the bright side, I might get a new pair of snazzy spectacles out of this!

Alright, maybe some of you (or all of you) weren't actually that enthusiastic about wearing a pair of glasses.

The funny thing with the above scenario though is that we tend not to ask whether going to the optometrists is necessary, I mean after all, it's their job and livelihood, they should definitely know what's best for our eyes. We tend to follow the norm and simply trust the optometrists' judgment and that they have our best interests at heart. As a result the majority of us end up being taken for a joy ride on the spectacle mill where we end up going for yearly or bi-yearly checkups and end up purchasing spectacles for the rest of our lives (we gotta make the most of our employee benefits right!)

More often than not however, going on this cycle isn't necessary, and eyesight can be corrected by using a few simple and easy exercises that some optometrists don't want you to know about; sometimes, they don't even know they exist or simply pretend they don't. We don't claim everything laid out here will correct 100% of all eye problems (if anyone ever claims to fix everything they're most likely trying to sell you something!), but the blueprint presented here will most certainly improve your vision to a significant extent.

Some optometrists are really good and you may find your prescription lessening over time instead of getting stronger. They may even advise you on certain eye exercises and the effects eye strain has on your eye during everyday life and during eye exams (more to come later!).

THE TRUTH ABOUT LASIK SURGERY

Well we've covered the traditional way of dealing with eyesight issues, now that leaves us with the more modern and recent approach to it, LASIK or commonly known as laser eye surgery.

Sometimes, LASIK surgery is prescribed, a very expensive procedure which, just as with most corrective procedures has its own risks. The only issue I see here with LASIK surgery (excuse the pun – you'll get used to them by the end of the book, they're spread all throughout) is that it's just like putting a band-aid over a very deep cut which actually needs stitches. The eye surgery does not deal with the root cause, it merely leaves a band-aid over it which will eventually peel off and reveal the root causes that have been lurking underneath the whole time. You might be wondering what the root cause is, well you'll have to read on to find out!

I strongly believe laser eye surgery should only be a last resort option only due to the high risks that are posed, I highly advise those that I consult to exercise all options before going down this route as high risks are attached to it.

How laser eye surgery works is that a laser is used to reshape your cornea, and thus corrects any problems your eye or eyes might have focusing correctly. It is specifically designed to treat myopia (near-sightedness), hyperopia (far-sightedness) and astigmatism (a problem with focusing due to the shape of the eye).

THE RISKS OF LASIK SURGERY

Dry eyes

Developing dry eyes is very common after having this procedure. This often lasts for up to six months, and one would need eye medication during this period. Sometimes, however, it persists, and a follow-up procedure might be necessary to correct this state of affairs.

Haloes, glares and double vision

Many patients notice haloes around an object and find that they suddenly have double vision or even at times notice a glare after the procedure. Some patients also find that their sight in dim light is impaired to a greater degree than what it was before they had opted for surgery.

Problems with the eye flap

The eye flap is cut and put to the side during the surgery. Often, when it is put back, it can grow abnormally and this leads to problems such as infections that occur and eyes that tear more than what is usual.

Astigmatism

At times, when the tissue has been removed unevenly, astigmatism could occur, leading to the patient having to wear corrective eyeglasses or having to undergo corrective surgery.

Vision returns to where it was before the procedure

In some instances, the eye adjusts to its previous form. There are a number of reasons this might occur, e.g. pregnancy, the wound healing abnormally or even an imbalance in the patient's hormones.

Overcorrections or under-corrections

The surgeon may have removed too much or too little tissue. The patient might end up having to undergo another bout of surgery to correct this, although it is more difficult to correct overcorrections.

Loss of vision

Although rare, some patients have had a loss of vision due to this procedure.

It is recommended that one does their homework and researches laser therapy before embarking on this method of eye correction, and ENSURE that you are a good candidate before undergoing it (yes, there are good and bad candidates for this surgery!). Besides, why would you want to take unwarranted risks without exploring other options first?

Most people tend to opt for what is perceived as the easiest solution to the problem in the short-term but might not necessarily be beneficial for the long-term. Read on for the long-term options available in your arsenal!

CHAPTER 3 – HOW CAN 'EYE' SEE?

This chapter covers how our eyes work and how we have this 'superpower' we call vision, I recommend reading this chapter to help you understand how and why *The 20/20 Vision Blueprint* will improve your vision. However, if you ain't got no time for that, please feel free to jump to *Chapter 5 – 10 Eyesight Enhancing (E²) Exercises* on page 23 which starts with the eye exercises you can start doing right now.

BEYEOLOGY 101

Alright! For those of you hanging around, let's head down memory lane to biology class. To first understand how sight works, we need to understand the structure of the eye.

Please take 20 seconds to view and study the diagram on the next page, start from the right of the image (front of the eyeball where the cornea is) and gradually work your way to the left of the image (finishing at the back of the eyeball where the optic nerve is).

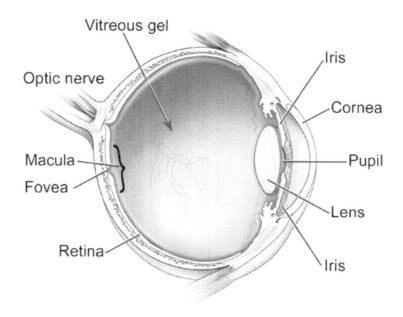

Image Courtesy of National Eye Institute

Beginning from the front of the eyeball, we will work our way towards the back explaining each part of the eye and their corresponding roles (feel free to refer back to the diagram as each part is explained):

The cornea is transparent and covers the front of the eye. It allows light in and acts as the first point of contact for light.

The iris (circle within the eye that determines your eye color) sits directly behind the cornea and is a ring of muscles that can contract or expand. The iris therefore regulates the size of your pupil depending on immediate lighting conditions and other factors.

The pupil - the black, inner circle of your eye is right in the middle of your iris. By contracting or expanding, it determines the amount of light that enters into your eye.

The sclera is the 'white of the eye' and its function is to protect the inner part of the eye.

The lens situated directly behind the pupil, reflects incoming light onto the retina.

The vitreous humor is a clear gel that makes up the largest part of your inner eyeball. It enables the eye to maintain its round shape (don't tell the eye that!)

The retina is a membrane (similar to a thin layer of tissue) which lines the inner surface of the eye. Its function is to take any incoming light and transform it into nerve signals.

The rods and cones are photoreceptors found in the retina, these two are the top dogs that convert light into nerve signals which your brain then processes. The rods and cones are very specialized; rods do the majority of the work in dark environments whilst cones do their share of work in lighter environments.

If you've ever wondered why it takes a while for our eyes to adjust when we enter a dark room (i.e. cinemas) it's because the cones in your retina are firing off while the rods are taking their sweet ass time to wake up and get to work.

Moving on…

The fovea is a very small spot which is found in the center of the retina. It helps to focus light rays to give you a crisp, sharp image (or a blurry, distorted one if it isn't doing its job properly).

The optic nerve is a bundle of nerve cells. Their purpose is to carry messages (nerve signals) sent from the eye to the brain, where the images are then processed to produce images which you see!

The macula is a small yet highly sensitive part of the retina. It is responsible for our central vision which allows us to see color, shapes and details clearly.

EYEING IT ALL UP!

The process whereby we see images can be summed up as follows:

1. Light passes through the **cornea** which bends the light rays so that it passes through the **pupil** (the black, center part of the eye) which is in the center of the **iris**.

2. The light then passes through the **lens** which 'accommodates' the ray of light by helping adjust the focus on both far and near objects so images are perceived clearly and sharply.

3. From here, the light rays pass through the vitreous gel and are focused so they reach the **retina**.

4. The **retina** then transforms the light rays into light impulses and nerve signals and sends them to the **optic nerve**. The **optic nerve** couriers these signals and impulses to the brain which then processes these signals into the images that we see!

Viola! That was simple enough wasn't it? The process is actually much more complex than those four steps but the basic premise holds. Eyesight problems usually occur when something goes wrong during one or more stages of the process.

Possible issues could include the scarring of the lenses or even an irregularity regarding the thickening of the cornea. But eye problems can start very small and quickly escalate out of control; this is commonly seen in people experiencing weeks or months of eye strain which then experience a sharp decline in vision or even from people being exposed to bright, harsh light rays for short periods of time.

CHAPTER 4 - THE #1 THING RESTRAINING YOU FROM ENHANCED VISION

There are many reasons our eyesight lets us down, but many are entirely preventable if we take the time to put in a little bit of effort. In the long run, nobody wants to really have eye surgery or wear spectacles or contacts for the rest of their lives: it costs a lot of money, can be time consuming, and in many instances a pain!

Don't tell me you've never forgotten to bring your glasses somewhere! Just think of all the time you've spent in the past trying to find your spectacles. Those frantic moments searching tirelessly for your spectacles whilst you continuously repeat to yourself "Where did I put them?!" well you can forget about that soon enough. :)

Let's take a look at some of the things that causes bad eyesight. There are many, however we will focus on the most common ones.

Eyestrain

When reading or working at your computer for long periods of time, this puts a lot of strain on your eyes. This strain usually leads to

16

headaches, dry eyes, eye fatigue, possible double vision, and, in many cases, near-sightedness! This is the NUMBER ONE THING you want to avoid if you want better vision.

You can clearly feel it (unless you've spent so much time with your eyes strained you've acclimatized to it) when you're reading things for a long period of time. There is a sense of droopiness and sometimes even blurry vision from the constant strain. We will dive deep into ways to prevent and lessen eye strain in the following chapter.

When your eyes have been strained for a period of time and you then go for an eye exam at the optometrists, your eye exam will be inaccurate and the prescription given to you will thus be inaccurate which can in turn harm your eyes.

THE THREE STOOGES

Apart from eyestrain these are the three other main factors hurting our vision:

1. Lack of nutrient-dense and whole foods

You may have been told to eat your vegetables when you were young, and this was for good reason! Proper nutrition is not only necessary for a healthy body and mind, but for healthy eyesight as well. This is really important as eyesight does not only depend on the eye and the corresponding muscles for good eyesight.

As explained earlier as to how vision works, the last step was the most important. A quick refresher for those who were writing notes during class – the last step involved the nerve signals and light impulses produced by the retina being sent to the brain, these signals and impulses were then processed to produce the images we see.

It doesn't matter how perfect your eye and the corresponding muscles are if your brain can't process the signals that are sent to it. The ability to which your brain functions and creates the grooves and ease of access to the neural pathways for processing these signals is highly dependent on having the nutrients it needs to do its job. This also relates highly to getting enough sleep so your brain can function properly, you would be surprised at the amount of clients I have that come to me that are functioning off five hours of sleep and have started to notice their vision deteriorating. The first thing I do is get them to start sleeping more and they notice remarkable improvements in their vision.

2. Aging

Nobody can stop the signs of aging! You can get Botox, have a facelift or try human growth hormone treatment, but the fact is, you can only change the outward signs of aging. Reversing the process is currently not possible in this day and age, but it's definitely possible to slow the process down by treating yourself right and taking the right precautionary measures.

3. Wearing your corrective eyewear all the time

Your eye has muscles that need exercise. By constantly wearing your spectacles or contacts, you're allowing these muscles to slack off and they never get a chance to exercise and stay well conditioned and thus end up deteriorating. This is the case for anything in life, whatever isn't growing or being maintained begins to atrophy and deteriorate. Think of any relationship, job or even your health in the past to the present and see how this concept relates. Your eyesight is no different.

This concept was clearly demonstrated in a fifteen year study done on how bras actually make women's breasts sag more because the muscles of the breast get reliant on the bras to lift them up so they weaken! This study was released in 2013, by the University of Franche-Comte if you are interested about it, consult Dr. Google. Another point to consider is how many times you've received exactly the same prescription for your eyes two times in a row? I'm willing to put money down that this is a rare occurrence for you.

6 COMMON EYE ISSUES

Below are six of the most common issues we face in today's society in regards to eyesight.

1. Strabismus, or as it is more often referred to, being cross-eyed

This often leads to frequent rubbing of the eyes and squinting to see properly. Most often, doctors recommend corrective eye surgery, but it is actually possible to correct this issue with certain eye exercises. This is quite prevalent with children in today's day and age.

2. Far-sightedness

This is a problem whereby the light rays which enter the eye are bent incorrectly. It causes blurred vision when you try to focus on something nearby.

3. Night blindness

As the condition states, this is where a person has problems with seeing correctly in dim light conditions.

4. Change in eyesight due to diabetes

Diabetes seems to be an illness of our times, and can have a real debilitating effect on our vision. The high blood sugar levels that people with diabetes have, can cause the lens of the eye to swell, and this can cause eyesight problems.

5. Glaucoma

This is a condition whereby there is an increase in pressure within the eye which causes damage to the optic nerve.

6. Astigmatism

An eye which has this problem is not round, like a normal eye, but shaped like a football. This causes problems with focusing correctly, and may result in either farsightedness or nearsightedness.

These are some of the most common eye issues we face in today's society however in later chapters we will touch more on them with preventative care and discuss further eye problems. Relating back to one of the three stooges, we have:

AGE RELATED EYE PROBLEMS

A person's eyesight is by no means static; it is something that, unfortunately, or fortunately, changes over time. It's quite common for someone to have perfect eyesight their whole lives, but as they age, they find they can no longer clearly see while reading or performing certain tasks. Even people who are nearsighted can experience this problem as they wear glasses or contact lenses that are supposed to help.

This phenomenon is called Presbyopia and usually comes into play when one passes the age of forty. It is thus regarded as a typically age-related process.

There are changes which occur within the lens' proteins that make the lens less elastic and harder over a period of time; in effect the lens becomes less flexible. Changes that are related to the aging process also affect the muscle fibers that surround the lens. Because the eye is now less elastic, it finds it harder to focus on objects which are close to you.

Cataracts

Of course, another problem regarding the eyes which is mostly age-related is cataracts, a clouding of the lens, which is usually removed by means of a surgical procedure. The clouding occurs as a result of the lens' protein clumping together and this is suspected to be caused by smoking, diabetes or through other means such as simple wear and tear (good news is that we can 'perform' maintenance on our eyes to take care of that wear and tear).

Glaucoma

Glaucoma is another common issue that is caused by damage done to the eye's optic nerve and is related to the pressure placed on the optic nerve. This is an eye problem which tends to be regarded as age-related.

Macular Degeneration

Another eye defect related to age (prevalent mainly in people over 50) is age-related macular degeneration (AMD). The macula becomes damaged and, in some cases loss of sight occurs over a short period, while in others it is a process that takes place over a very long period. It is suspected that those who are at a higher risk of AMD are smokers or those who have a family history of the disease.

No person can stop the effects of aging, but you can limit the effects by doing a few simple exercises on a regular basis! All it costs is a little time and effort, and it is something you can do for the rest of your life for free so let's get to it shall we.

CHAPTER 5 - 10 EYESIGHT ENHANCING (E²) EXERCISES

We have now had a look at facts about the eyes, how vision works, the main reason our vision deteriorates and some of the different kinds of eye problems out there (unless you skipped to this chapter!). Now let's get down to the fun stuff, the E² exercises you've been waiting for.

THE BATES METHOD

The Bates Method of training your eyes and the corresponding exercises outlined here were designed by William Bates. If we check out this man's credentials (I'm not talking about the size of his wallet); he was an ophthalmologist a.k.a. a surgeon – who was well regarded by his peers. He was renowned for being a brilliant man, as he had not only discovered the properties of adrenaline, but had also pioneered an ear operation to reverse deafness, an operation which is still carried out to this day.

No doubt Bates was a very learned and clever man. But his

reputation all changed once he started working on techniques that could correct eyesight. These techniques and exercises included correcting everything from lazy eye to farsightedness to reversing the effects of age-related eye problems, you name it, he studied it and documented it all for us to use. This, as you could imagine, did not sit too well with his peers, especially for his era (late 1800's and early 1900's).

His peers ridiculed him and attempted to discredit his work within the scientific community. Nevertheless, he carried on with his work and these exercises, as advocated by him, are still with us to this very day, although very few people in the industry would recommend you try them, let alone tell you about them.

The Bates Method was strongly supported by Aldous Huxley (a British author most well-known for Brave New World):

"Within a couple of months I was reading without spectacles and, what was better still, without strain and fatigue… At the present time, my vision, though very far from normal, is about twice as good as it used to be when I wore spectacles" – Aldous Huxley

All the E² Exercises mentioned are to be done with no corrective eyewear so it is highly suggested the exercise be done in the morning or before bed if you wear contacts, otherwise throw your glasses to the side whilst doing the exercises. As you read along try the exercises at least once, don't worry about memorizing how to do it all, when you reach the end of the book you can get the free bonuses that includes the 20/20 Vision Blueprint worksheets as well as a resource cheat sheet and book summary notes with all the exercises and instructions.

> **TIP:** As you do the exercises, try to focus on deep breathing and feeling the motion and eyes as you do it. Consciously relax them and be mindful of how you are breathing (you want deep and slow, not sharp and short!).

PALMING

This is an extremely easy exercise to do!

Simply cover your eyes with both palms, letting your fingers cross each other as they rest on your forehead. Don't place excessive pressure on your eyes with your palms, and make sure your eye sockets are covered so that very little to NO light enters past your hands.

You can do this exercise while sitting up straight with your arms supported, or while lying down with your feet on the floor, whichever is the most comfortable position for you! Keep your neck and shoulder muscles relaxed.

How long should you do this for? Well, that depends on you! Try it for 2 minutes and then ask yourself how you feel. If you feel calm, rested and happy, then you can do it for less otherwise keep going and do your best to relax and focus on your breath. Let your body and daily schedule set the pace!

You might be wondering: "how frequently should I do this?" and the answers as often as you can throughout the day! If you have a few minutes while waiting for the coffee maker, do it! Sitting at a bus stop? Do it! It can be done anywhere, for any length of time, for as often as you wish, but preferably spread it out throughout the day.

Just doing it for the count of ten to fifteen slow breaths helps relieve eye strain (the #1 killer of good eyesight). Some of you might think you could look silly doing this but if anyone asks what on earth you're doing, just say you're making a wish and that'll get a good laugh out of both of you.

It's not the length of time you palm for that makes a difference, but rather the frequency with which you do it that counts!

TIP: Open your eyes once you've placed your hands over your eye sockets to see if any light is coming in, if there is light coming in adjust your hands so that they are blocking the incoming light then close your eyes and continue with the palming.

Why It Works

The palming method allows your eyes to have a rest and eases any eyestrain you may be experiencing and it also allows your body and mind to take a rest thus reducing any stress you may be experiencing.

THE SWAY

This is exactly what the title suggests: a rhythmic swaying from side to side (think of the push and pulls you experience as you stand on a train that is constantly starting and stopping). This is highly recommended after palming as your eyes and mind are most relaxed after palming.

How it's done:

1. Stand in a relaxed position with your feet about shoulder width apart and hands relaxed by your side.

2. Gently, start swaying from side to side placing your weight on the foot of the side you are swaying towards so it's supporting you.
   Let the heel of the non-supporting foot lift away from the floor slightly if you can keep your balance whilst doing so. Use your hands to balance yourself as you sway if you need to otherwise let them hang free.

3. While you are swaying, focus your eyes on a point or object far away from you (don't worry if you can't see it clearly), the distance should be at least 5 feet away from you and should be no more than 20 feet.

4. Once you have a steady focus, try closing your eyes and carry on with the movement, paying attention to the sounds around you whilst breathing slowly.

5. When you are feeling more relaxed as you continue swaying open your eyes again and focus on the object you picked earlier. You might notice that features nearer to you seem to be swaying as well, but keep your focus on that object you picked!

This exercise is easier for people who have good eyesight, but practice, practice, practice. The more you do it, the easier it gets! The best part about this exercise is the instant improvements you can notice

"The world moves. Let it move. All objects move if you let them. Do not interfere with this movement, or try to stop it. This cannot be done without an effort which impairs the efficiency of the eye and mind." - W. Bates: Better Eyesight Magazines, July 1920

THE SWINGS

There are four different variations of the swing, and many people actually combine them or find their own variation. As long as the basic principles are adhered to feel free to experiment as it brings the same results.

The Long Swing

For this exercise you need a ruler or any other item that is similar in length, the item should be light and easy to handle.

Hold the item in front of you with both hands so it is vertical to the ground and hold it at an arm's length away from you. Begin swaying, as the previous exercise explained, but with one exception: twist your body and feet to the left or the right then repeat the motion. Remember to keep your eyes on the ruler!

If, at some point, you start feeling dizzy or uncomfortable, stop.

Do some palming until the sensation passes, and carry on again from there. Try this exercise for 1-2 minutes, more or less depending on how comfortable you feel doing the exercise which means if your eyes start to strain or you become dizzy, chill out and palm out for a bit.

TIP: You don't have to twist your body that far, 90 degrees to the left or right is adequate otherwise whatever is most comfortable for you.

The Head Swing

The head swing can be done anywhere, but many people find it more difficult than the long swing because it involves turning your neck and not your feet and body. It's an exercise which is similar to the long swing.

Keep your eyes as relaxed as possible while doing this exercise.

For this exercise, you need to turn your head from side to side. Imagine watching bicycles go past you or that your nose is the size of Pinocchio after telling one too many lies and you're watching the tip of your nose as you swing your head left to right and back again.

We are aiming to move in a smooth motion here, we don't want a jerky movement. Don't stop the head movement to consciously focus on any one thing! As before, do this for as long as you feel comfortable, a good starting point is 2 to 3 minutes.

Try out your own variations of this, but remember to keep those eyes relaxed and do not strain to focus your eyes!

The Prayer Swing

This is very similar to the head swing, but, you keep the eyes closed!

1. Sit down at a desk or table.

2. Place your elbows on the desk or table and clasp your hands together as if you're praying.

3. Close your eyes, and keep your eyes relaxed and facing straight forward throughout the exercise.

4. Turn your head as you would in the head swing exercise. Remember, not to focus or strain your eyes here, keep them as relaxed as possible.

Sunning

The easiest way to practice this method is by using a lamp, preferably an anglepoise lamp such as the one below. I have provided resources at the end of this book in the bonus section which lists the specific items I use and recommend for these exercises so don't fret.

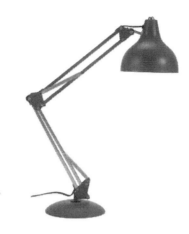

These desk lamps are quite handy for this exercise as you can turn them to different angles. If you don't have one that's all good, we can get innovative! Any lamp that can shine light at your face will easily do.

The sun is the best source of light for this exercise, but it can be a little too bright at certain times during the day and, during winter, sunlight might be something that is a little difficult to come by.

Make sure you are sitting somewhere which is comfortable when you perform sunning; this makes it easier to do some palming after you have completed the sunning exercise which is highly recommended.

Get Some of That Vitamin D!

To perform sunning:

1. Sit with your eyes closed with the light shining directly on your face – you can adjust the distance until it's at a comfortable temperature for you. You should experience pleasant warmth

from the light.

2. Keeping your eyes closed and looking straight ahead, slowly turn your head from side to side. Your eyes need to stay "looking ahead" the whole time and not move.

3. As you turn your head, one side will be shadowed from the light, the other will be facing the light.

Why It Works

Sunning with your eyes closed allows the retina to get used to a range of bright lights so that the entire range can be tolerated without ill effect on the eyes. This is done by turning left to right and allowing the broad range of brightness emitting from the lamp to land on your eyelids.

TIP: If your eyes tend to move around, go even slower! The aim is to   keep them still here. Perform sunning for a maximum of three minutes   then stop and perform the palming exercise until your eyes have   'calmed' down and feel rested. If you want to use the sun as a source   of light, please only do so during sunrise or sunset as the UV rays emitted from the sun are weakest during these points of the day.

PINHOLE GLASSES

Before we look at pinhole glasses and their benefits, we first need to know what they are, exactly. Basically, they look like sunglasses, except the lenses are black and aren't transparent. They also have a myriad of tiny holes in them.

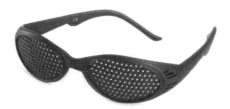

This may seem to be a really cool (or odd) look to some people, but these glasses do, in fact, have the added benefit of helping to improve your eyesight!

How do they work?

In a nutshell, each hole allows light to enter your eye and focus on your retina as a very narrow beam of light increasing depth of field. Essentially it exercises your retina on a broader spectrum thus transferring benefits over to your normal daily activities.

Because this breaks down the beam of light so it isn't just one large beam of light (as is normal) you have a lot of smaller rays penetrating your eye which ends up forming the same image that passes through different points on your retina.

At first, the resulting image may be a little blurry, especially around the edges, but with continued use and the exercises mentioned above you will definitely see a marked improvement in images.

Please do not use these glasses while driving or doing other activities which require functioning vision for safety reasons, as it does reduce your peripheral vision. They can be used to watch TV or reading and it is suggested you slowly 'wear them in' before you wear them for extended periods of time.

Two simple exercises to do with pinhole exercises is to imagine a box, with your eyes go to each of the four corners of the box in a clockwise direction 10 times, then reverse it to go in an anti-clockwise direction 10 times. After that, move your eyes left to right 10 times then repeat going from right to left.

EYE FIXATION

Imagine drawing a line down the center of your forehead and nose, now; draw another line across the bottom of your eyebrows. These two imaginary lines should form a plus sign (+).

Now, turn both eyes inward and look at that spot for a few seconds. A tip is to use your finger and watch the tip of your finger as you bring it closer to your face until it touches the spot where the two lines would cross.

Hold this position for ten seconds then slowly increase this period as you practice. This is excellent for exercising the eye muscles, make sure not to strain too hard whilst doing this exercise.

ROLLING EYE MOVEMENTS (FOR EYE MUSCLES)

Imagine a horizontal figure 8 (∞). Now, only using your eyes, trace the outline of this figure seven times. Do the exercise slowly and smoothly.

When you are done, repeat the exercise, this time tracing the outline of a normal figure 8. Again, do this in a slow and controlled manner so that all eye muscles are exercised and to ensure they aren't strained during the exercise. This exercise can be done with your eyes closed or open, whichever you find easiest to visualize the figure 8's with is recommended.

Blink rapidly or do some palming afterwards so that you can relax the eyes and let them 'cool' down.

PREVENTING EYE FATIGUE WHILE READING

Reading or staring at a computer screen, laptop, kindle or iPad for long periods of time are known to cause stress and strain on the eyes. This is inevitable in today's world as these gadgets are used for our livelihood and entertainment. Fortunately, the trick to preventing strain and eye fatigue whilst using these tools is easy. Just by following a few easy steps, you can limit the damage caused from using these instruments.

What is eyestrain or eye fatigue?

Simply put, it's when you've been reading for a long period of time and in turn have been concentrating on something that is in close proximity to you. The eyes as a result may get tired, itchy, and dry or you might even experience a slight burning sensation.

How to prevent it:

If you're working on a computer, make sure the screen is about 20 to 25 inches away and that the screen is slightly lower than your field of vision. In essence, you want to be looking at the screen from a slightly downwards angle, slightly tucking your chin into your body.

- Make sure the screen is clean (smudges can be irritable on the eye) and that minimal glare is coming off the screen.

- Use the **20/20/20 rule** - for every 20 minutes you spend reading or working, look at an object 20 feet away from you (this can be anything, just focus on a point roughly 20 feet from you), for approximately 20 seconds.

- Take regular breaks! Stand up, go outside, make some coffee or have a chat to someone. Do anything that gets you away from the screen or book you might be reading for a few minutes if you have been at it for over an hour.

- This one sounds silly, but remember to blink! Your eyes need fluid to prevent them from drying out and lubrication of your eyes is done through blinking. This is actually a common issue when people are focusing too hard for extended periods of time.

- Use eye drops if you feel your eyes start feeling dry. This is only necessary for those who chronically experience dry eyes; the best solution here is to drink more water.

- If you forgot to blink or use eye drops and your eyes are feeling dry, wet a washcloth with warm water, wring it out, close your eyes, lay back, and cover your face and eyes with the washcloth.

- If you're working indoors in dry conditions where there isn't good air flow consider using a humidifier.

These steps are mostly common sense, but we often forget about incorporating them. It's crucial that you pick two of the suggested active approaches and undertake it for at least seven days; you will easily find yourself doing them habitually after these seven days and your eyes will be better for it!

CHAPTER 6 - EYE-WATERING FOODS

LIFESTYLE IMPROVEMENTS

Now that we've covered the chapter on exercises (I hope you tried each exercise at least once by now, if not please go back and do the ones you haven't managed to do yet!), we will dive deeper into the next level of improving our eyesight and that starts with our food. You are what you eat, eat garbage and you will feel and function like garbage.

In general, it is advised that one eats a balanced diet, including all components, i.e. red meat, poultry, fish, and a wide range of fruit and vegetables.

Your eyes, like the rest of your body, is dependent on the nutrients and vitamins contained in food, and a proper, healthy eating plan is thus important to ensure optimal eyesight and in many cases aid in the reversal of eyesight issues.

What's Up Doc?

Remember when you were small and you were told to eat carrots because they were good for your eyes? Well, that's a myth! Although vegetables, which are rich in vitamins and minerals, do indeed help your eyesight, carrots don't directly enhance your vision, this myth started due to British propaganda in World War II. An article was printed in the British press stating that the Royal Air Force pilots had exceptional night vision due to eating excess carrots that enhanced their night time vision. They tied this into why the pilots had such great success detecting enemy bombers when in fact they had just been using new technology termed the Airborne Interception Radar to detect enemy bombers with greater precision and accuracy.

Carrots do help with your night vision to a certain degree as they contain beta-carotene which your liver turns into Vitamin A. Vitamin A is a necessary precursor for your eyes to see in dim light but this doesn't directly translate to better vision overall, Vitamin A can be found in your **sweet potatoes, carrots, dark leafy greens, apricots, mango and cantaloupe.**

Lutein Fat Foods

Lutein is what forms pigments in the macula and is necessary to help prevent macular degeneration which is one of the leading causes of eye loss, especially in the elderly. Foods which are rich in lutein include your **green, leafy vegetables** such as **broccoli, spinach** and **kale**.

Omega-3 Fatty Acids

Foods that are rich in Omega-3 fatty acids, such as tuna, sardines and salmon are extremely important for your eye health as the essential fatty acids in them are necessary for the production of the water and oil layers of the tear film which maintains the transparency and health of your cornea. One of the most important Omega-3 fatty acids is Docosahexaenoic Acid (DHA). DHA makes up 93% of the Omega-3 acids in the eye, and it has been proven through studies that when a mother has had an above average intake of this essential acid while pregnant, the child tends to have better eyesight than other children which weren't provided as much DHA.

In short, to improve your vision to the best of your ability, make sure you get enough DHA in your diet, together with the eye exercises described, this is a sure way of getting you on the right track. Fish oil supplements are a highly recommended supplement for overall general health as well as eyesight if you don't eat fish often.

Next time you think of having a barbeque, think of smoking up some fish!

Turn On The Waterfalls!

Dry eyes are not only caused by prolonged periods of eye strain, but also by free radicals which are the result of smoking, a poor diet, aging, excess alcohol, chronic stress or certain medications. A diet which is rich in a variety of vegetables, especially **leafy vegetables** such as **kale, spinach** or **chard** helps combat this, as well as fruits such as a variety of different **berries** and **cherries**.

Three juicing recipes are included below for those who don't have the time or inclination to eat all these fruit and vegetables.

One of the best methods for hydrating dry and tired eyes is water! Yes, we hear about water and its benefits everywhere these days, but did you know that an average person comprises 65% of water?

That's more than half our body composition! The Institute of Medicine recommends a fluid intake of roughly 100 ounces (13 glasses) for men and 75 ounces (9 glasses) for women a day. Water is not just a necessity to keep us from dehydrating, it's the means by which our body flushes out toxins and carries essential nutrients to the cells in our body. On top of that it ensures our eyes have a nice healthy, moist environment to function properly.

Now, not all people tend to drink that much water in today's age because of all the other options available, but it is highly, highly recommended you begin substituting the sodas or beers for a few glasses of water wherever possible. For those who want to start drinking more water but find the taste too dull, I've provided a few recipes for water infusions. Try one of these recipes out, and I'm sure you'll try them all!

3 INSTANT AND DELICIOUS JUICING RECIPES THAT SUPERCHARGE YOUR VISION

1. Bright eyes

2 Apples

1/4 chunk of medium sized carrot

1/2 stick of Celery

1 large handful of mixed green leaves – watercress, kale, parsley, spinach or any other green leafy vegetables you have on hand

1 inch slice Cucumber

1/2 inch Broccoli stem

1/4 inch slice unpeeled raw Beetroot

1/4 inch slice Zucchini (courgette)

1 small piece of Lemon – preferably, wax-free with rind on

1/4 inch slice Ginger

Add all the ingredients together in a juicer and throw some ice cubes in!

2. Pineapple Surprise

3/4 Medium Pineapple

3 cm chunk of Broccoli Stem

2 cm Fresh Ginger Root chunk

Juice everything together and add ice cubes. This is a really refreshing drink for a hot summer's day.

3. Carrot Twist

2 Apples

1/2 Beetroot

2 small Carrots

1 small Parsnip

1/4 lemon (keep the peel on if it has not been waxed, or scrub it off.)

Juice all ingredients together, and add ice cubes if you would like.

3 SIMPLE INFUSED WATER CONCOCTIONS YOU'RE MISSING OUT ON

Infused water is simply water that has fruits, herbs or spices added to it. The water is then left to stand so that the properties of the ingredients can infuse into the water (usually overnight) to be drunk the next day. Here are a few ingredient combinations.

1. Apple/Cinnamon Infusion

1/4 apple, finely sliced with a stick of Cinnamon.

Add the ingredients to a liter of water, leave it overnight, and enjoy in the morning.

2. Mango and Mint (M&M)

2 sprigs of mint and ½ a mango peeled and chopped.

Add ingredients to a liter of water and leave overnight.

3. Mixed Herbs

This is incredibly easy!

Pick whatever herbs you have available, crush the leaves slightly, and add them to a liter of water. Allow the infusion to stand overnight.

TIP: With any of the above infused water recipes, allow at least five hours before drinking to ensure ingredients have been steeped long enough. Herbs should be slightly crushed and fruit sliced, diced or chunky!

CHAPTER 7 - PREVENTION IS CHEAPER THAN TREATMENT!

Prevention is always better than cure! So what can you, as someone who has good eyesight do to prevent it from going south? Or, if your vision has deteriorated in some way, what can you do to prevent it going further south?

LOOK OUT FOR THESE!

Well, in addition to doing the exercises listed, the following points must be considered:

Prolonged periods of staring at your computer screen, smartphone, kindle, etc

Give your eyes a break on a consistent basis – remember 20/20/20! Also consider upgrading your old computer monitors if you still have them to the newer flat screens as they prevent or reduce glare drastically. Optionally position your computer screen so it has reduced glare. While using the computer you can also enlarge text by holding down the 'Ctrl' key and scrolling up with the mouse wheel.

Read **BIGGER** print

On your Kindle you can adjust the size of the font and letterings! Also try using a low magnitude magnifying glass for small print such as when reading newspapers or other small print and you won't have to strain your eyes.

Aim air vents in car downwards instead of straight in the direction of your eyes

Constant air blown into your eyes can cause dryness in the eyes and ruin your vision.

The use of safety goggles

When doing any kind of work with the possibility of foreign objects penetrating your eyes, wear them. It may not look aesthetically pleasing or feel nice, but they are there for a reason!

Using eye drops too frequently

Your eyes can produce their own fluid; use eye drops only as necessary otherwise your eyes will gradually become more and more dependent on eye drops much like your eyes and corrective eyewear.

Rubbing your eyes frequently

If you frequently rub your eyes it can cause the blood vessels to rupture, especially if you are rubbing with force.

Watching television (or using any electronic device with a screen) in the dark

This can cause long term damage. Always make sure the room or electronic device has adequate lighting so your eyes don't have to strain whilst reading or watching.

Sunglasses

Wearing good quality sunglasses that protect against harmful UV rays during hours of the day when UV is the highest is strongly recommended.

Sleep

We might not realize this, but sleep deprivation is not only unhealthy for a myriad of things such as weight gain and weakened immune systems, but it's also a major cause of dry eyes, blurry vision and headaches. So get as much good quality sleep as you feel you need to feel refreshed and energized!

Smoking

There's a lot out there in terms of the negative effects smoking has on our bodies. In terms of vision it can accelerate the development of certain eye diseases such as macular degeneration, dry eyes and even diabetic retinopathy.

A poor diet

We've covered this point already but it's repeated here again because of how important it is. A quick recap: ensure your diet incorporates a large variety of fresh fruit, green leafy vegetables, meat, fish and poultry. These foods all aid in combatting eye degeneration.

Water

We need our daily intake to ensure the proper function and fluid-making ability of the eyes.

Ladies – limit your makeup!

Replace your eye makeup every few months (this is a good excuse to go shopping!), it helps prevent bacteria from developing in your makeup and getting into your eyes. Also try not to wear eye makeup for more than 8 hours and ensure you remove makeup completely before heading to bed.

ESSENTIAL VITAMINS AND CATARACTS

Cataracts are something which we associate with the elderly, but there are instances where other factors come into play, such congenital reasons (meaning you were born with them), some form as a result of prolonged steroid use, eye injuries or even smoking. However, more often than not, it is thought of as an age-related eye problem.

The chances of contracting this eye disease can, however, be lowered by following a balanced diet, as cataracts are mainly formed due to a lack of the proper nutrients in one's diet. Think in terms of foods rich in vitamins C (dark leafy greens, citrus fruits, tomatoes, broccoli) and E (almonds, raw seeds, spinach, raw seeds, kale, hazelnuts). The antioxidants found in them can reduce a person's risk of cataract development by sixty percent!

CHAPTTER 8 - TWO OVERPRESCRIBED DRUGS HOLDING YOU BACK FROM 20/20

What is scary in today's day and age is that so many prescribed drugs and even those you can buy at your regular drug store, may actually harm you or your eyesight. Yes, this is no joke! What's worse is the fact that some doctors, it would seem, are not even aware of the side effects some of these drugs have on our eyes, never mind the rest of our bodies, and if they do, they rarely tell us about them!

Have you ever thought about that? Have you ever asked them about the side effects of the little round objects they are often so eager to give to only get an answer which is vague and generic so they can hurry in the next patient? Very few of us even question the side effects, I mean the doctors are medical professionals and it's their job to help us, right? I highly suggest you draw your own conclusions and do your own research before ingesting any pills or drugs you're recommended. Google is awesome and will help you freely with this!

Below we have two of the most common drugs that are used daily by the public hurting our eyesight.

ANTIHISTAMINES

These seemingly innocuous pills can contribute to the formation of cataracts; worsen narrow-angle glaucoma, dry eyes and macular degeneration.

Did you know that there are natural antihistamines?

Some examples include: Caraway and Fennel seeds, Basil, Anise, Saffron, Parsley, Cardamon, and Echinacea.

Simply make a tea of their dried leaves, and drink, or, alternatively, many are available from health food shops in capsulated form.

ANTIBIOTICS

Have a sniffle, running eyes or maybe a bit of a cough? You might be suffering from a common cold.

If that's the case, your doctor would most probably prescribe you an antibiotic, yet, this is one of the most overprescribed medications there are, and to make matters worse, they are only effective when used for bacterial infections. They have no use whatsoever against viral infections, and the common cold, I'm sorry to tell you, is a viral infection!

Just how can antibiotics affect your eyesight adversely? Remember that antibiotics prescribed by doctors don't contain natural ingredients, as nobody can have a patent for a natural plant.

Some of the adverse effects of antibiotics pertaining to eye health are that they are all basically a synthetic form of penicillin. Penicillin can contribute to: increased light sensitivity, glaucoma, allergic conjunctivitis (when applied topically), retinal detachment, blurred vision, and even aid in the formation of cataracts in fetuses. There are quite a few nasty side effects with this one.

You might be wondering whether there are natural substitutions for this drug that traditionally, has been prescribed as the cure-all for most of the ailments suffered today. Of course there is!

Here are a few: raw honey, garlic, Echinacea, turmeric, olive leaf extract (available at many health food stores), and ginger.

A typical natural aid to the common cold: A tablespoon of honey, a good squeeze of lemon juice, a half teaspoon of crushed, fresh ginger and half a glass of warm water.

Stir it all together, and drink this a few times a day. Tasty, yet effective! The lemon juice gives the added dose of vitamin C necessary to help fight colds, and the honey also helps to soothe a sore throat. For those of you who like your medicine to have an added kick to it: add some whisky (only joking!).

There are many other types of medication prescribed for the common illnesses which are experienced in this day and age, but the aim here is to make you think and make informed choices about the things you are ingesting. Always ask the question:

'Is this medication necessary, and if so, what are the possible side effects?'

'Is there something else that can be prescribed or taken that would have less side effects?'

'What interaction effects will it have on me if used in conjunction with other medication I'm taking?'

We have covered quite a lot of ground, but consider this:

By taking these factors which we have discussed into account, one is sure to be doing your best in preventing any further eye problems.

CHAPTER 9 - ANCIENT AYURVEDIC EXERCISES AND CHINESE REMEDIES

Failing eyesight is not something that is unique to this day and age, in fact it's something which has been a problem since the dark ages and as a result has been addressed by some of the most ancient civilizations, such as those in India, China, and Tibet. Although we won't be discussing all of the techniques in great detail, a few of the best remedies and exercises in my own and other's experiences are presented here.

AYURVEDA

Ayurveda is one of the oldest holistic forms of healing and was developed thousands of years ago in India. It's a system of healing based on the belief that to be emotionally and physically well, your body, mind and spirit must be in a state of balance. As a result, Ayurvedic medicine promotes good health and does not fight disease, per se. It works on the premise of prevention rather than cure. It sounds a bit more appealing than the western paradigm doesn't it?

Instead of diagnosing the surface symptoms and directly treating them first, go straight to the core root of the problem and solve that instead. Ayurveda aims at promoting health and wellbeing so that you don't get ill in the first place. This is a bit of a turnaround from the mainstream thought processes.

The study of Ayurveda is in itself an art, and we could write a whole book about it, but for our purposes, we are going to look solely at its take on eyesight.

The Five Elements

According to the Ayurvedic view, there are five elements that concern the eyes: earth, air, fire, water and space, each one governs a different area, and has a unique function. To ensure optimum eye health, it is believed that all of these must be in balance, and one must take measures to ensure they are balanced. By taking care of your eyes, they believe you won't have to treat ailments because they won't occur in the first place. There are a few recommended Ayurverdic exercises and recipes which help to keep these elements balanced and in place.

THE AYURVEDIC TRIFECTA

1. Dry or Tired Eyes

Splash your face with lukewarm water in the mornings – about 10 to 15 times.

Drink fennel seed water daily – boil a teaspoon of fennel seeds with a cup of water until the volume of water has been reduced by half. Drink when the tea is cool.

TIP: Remember to strain the tea first so you aren't guzzling down fennel seeds!

2. Relieving Eyestrain

A variation of palming is recommended here. Rub your palms together for a few seconds so they heat up slightly. Place your palms over your eyes, without putting any pressure on the eye ball. Repeat this a few times for lengths of 2 to 3 minutes.

3. Strengthen Eye Muscles

Sit on the floor cross legged with your back comfortably straight, knees bent and legs crossed. Face directly ahead of you with your hands resting on your knees.

Start off by looking straight ahead. Refrain from moving your head during this exercise. Breathe deeply and slowly throughout this exercise and remember to relax, this can be done by just watching and following your breath. Listen to your body and feel it out.

Once you have yourself in position and you're quite relaxed, raise your eyes to the ceiling, hold this for 2 seconds then slowly transition to looking downwards at the floor for two seconds, and close your eyes for 2 seconds.

Open your eyes then shift your eyes to the left and hold it there for 2 seconds, then to the right and hold it there for 2 seconds.

Look straight ahead again and close your eyes for 10seconds.

Repeat this exercise 4 – 5 times.

The seconds provided for each movement can be altered to be longer or shorter, feel free to experiment with different lengths and don't get stuck on having to count each movement. Do what feels comfortable for you.

3 CHINESE HERBAL REMEDIES

The Ancient Chinese also believe in a holistic approach when it comes to the eyes. They have, over centuries, developed remedies that we can brew up in our own homes to help combat and remedy eye problems. If these remedies and herbs have been used for thousands of years, they've got to have some effect right? They would have gone out of fashion a long time ago if they didn't do anything!

These Chinese remedies consist mainly of brewed teas that are refreshing and tasty:

THE CHINESE TEAFECTA

1. Mulberry Leaf Tea

Who knew that mulberry leaves weren't only for silkworms?

Soak a handful of dried mulberry leaves in a cup full of hot water and let it brew for five minutes then drink up! This tea is said to improve dry eyes, headaches, and even helps combat dizziness. It's also purported to assist with allergies.

2. Green Tea

I think most of us know how good green tea is for us, and not to mention it's freely available at your local supermarket. A teaspoon of the tea with a cup of boiling water over is enough. This tea has so many anti-oxidant properties that there are too many to mention. However, as far as eyesight is concerned, they protect your eyes against glaucoma and other eye diseases such as macular degeneration.

3. Chrysanthemum Tea

Yes, we're talking about the flower that grows in your garden! The tea made from these flowers has long been used to treat dry and tired eyes. Next time you come home from a long day spent in front of a computer screen, try a cup of chrysanthemum tea; you might be surprised at how refreshed you'll feel afterwards. Chrysanthemum tea is available at most Chinese food stores.

TIBETAN EYE CHART

The Ancient Chinese and Indian cultures were not the only ancient cultures that were concerned with eye health. The ancient Tibetans devised a chart along with eye exercises geared towards improving eye conditions which is on the next page.

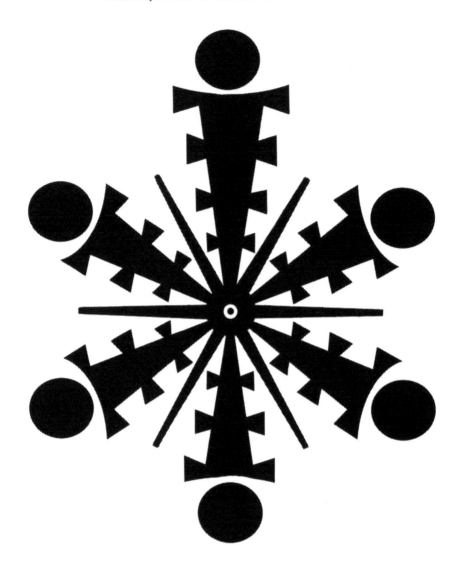

These exercises were devised specifically to strengthen the eye muscles and the optic nerve.

1. Start off by palming to get your eyes relaxed ('cold' or 'hot' palming will do).

2. Direct your eyes to the center of each dot on the outskirts of

the chart and move to the next dot in a clockwise direction.

3. Once you reach the starting dot, repeat Step 2 in an anticlockwise direction.

4. When you have reached the starting dot again. Direct your vision and move between the two circles at the 2 0'clock and 8 o'clock positions (top right and bottom left circles) slowly back and forth. Repeat this five times.

5. This time repeat Step 4 but with the 4 o'clock and 10 o'clock circles (top left and bottom right circles).

6. Once finished, blink rapidly for five seconds, and then repeat the palming technique.

You can do this whole exercise a few times (aim for three at first), but ensure you don't over-strain your eyes and keep your eyes as relaxed as possible.

CHAPTER 10 – CONCLUSION

This has been a lot of information to digest, yet we so often fail to remember that we should, and indeed could, be part of our own healing process; that today's society has become so dependent on what the "experts" say, that we so often forget that a few hundred years ago, all medication and methods of healing were 100% natural! Back then there were no 'magic' pills to pop to 'heal' almost every disease conceivable to man. Natural herbs, spice, and vegetables were the only ingredients in the healing remedies used at that time, and that, in many instances, easy exercises were used to help treat common eye problems.

Doctors at the time, treated their patients holistically, and usually looked at the causes of their problems, and did not only treat the symptoms of the illness or problem experienced. Each of us were seen as an individual entity, and our bodies and minds as a part of the same hole. In essence, they treated our minds, souls and bodies. These days, the symptoms are treated, and much of the medication or procedures prescribed have detrimental side effects.

The eyes, it is so often said, is the gateway to the soul, and very often the first thing we notice when looking at someone for the first time, and they need to be treated with the respect that they deserve. Does this not mean that we need to be aware of all the ways and means out there that can be used to look after them, to strengthen them, and to heal them? We need to be a part of the solution regarding the medical treatments we are given, and we need to be made aware of all the options available to us, both naturally and of a man-made nature, so that we can make informed decisions.

So many of our eye illnesses, can be 'fixed' using the natural means that have been detailed in this book, whether it is by changing our diet so that we follow a more healthy lifestyle, doing eye exercises to strengthen the different parts of the eye and improve their function, or natural herbs and medication that have no detrimental effect on either our eyesight or our general health.

Besides, the benefits of the lifestyle changes we can make do not only concern our eyes, but our general, overall, well-being as well! To add to this, most of these changes will save you money in the long run, not only on medical bills, but on your food bill as well, as cutting out pizzas and burgers from the local take-out store and replacing them with a healthy eating option, is guaranteed to save you quite a large amount of money in your monthly budget – money that can be used towards your yearly vacation, for example. This does not mean that we have to completely do without that lovely, cheese-oozing slice of pizza, but remember, moderation in all things!

The thing to remember when doing these eye exercises is

consistency. You cannot do them for a week and expect a miracle to happen almost overnight. No, they need to be done every day, in some instances more than once a day, over a long period of time – preferably for the rest of your life. They are not only aimed to help you improve your eyes, they are there to keep your vision functioning optimally! So, the more you do them, the longer you do them, the better your eyesight will become. And please remember: these exercises are to be done without spectacles or contact lenses! Wearing them while doing the exercises would defeat the purpose.

The herbs that are mentioned have been used for thousands of years, and have been proven to be effective. It might seem strange, at first, concocting teas to drink, but, as with most things in life, if you do something often enough, over time, it becomes a habit, and once it is a habit, it has the potential to become a lifelong way of life. Thus, perseverance will result in long term benefits that could very well last until the day you die.

Where children are concerned, by introducing the exercises as a game will guarantee a healthy habit that will last a lifetime, and they will most probably end up doing them without even thinking about it. But to start off, make it fun, something the family can do together, so that they understand that they are not 'weird', but that good eye practice is a way of life, and not something that suddenly happens the day the optometrist tells them that they need glasses.

The saying *'prevention is better than cure'* is most certainly applicable as far as our eyes are concerned. Even if you have perfect, 20/20 vision, you can still reap the benefit of following the exercises, lifestyle changes and drinking the herbal teas and juices described. It is by far easier to maintain something than to correct it.

If you decide to follow the exercises described here, please remember that Rome was not built in a day and that the exercises need to be done daily to ensure optimum effectiveness. Get your free bonus pack at the end of the book for the 20/20 Vision Blueprint and 21 day program that will ensure your success!

Remember: In no way is it advised to treat your eyes, or eye-care specialists with disdain! The aim of this book is to inform its reader of an alternative, natural approach to eye care, so that you can make informed decisions regarding the subject, but also take an active role in its treatment. If you wear glasses currently and feel they may be too strong, please go see your optometrist about lowering your prescription. Also ensure to perform the palming exercise before heading in to make sure your eyes aren't straining when you undertake the eye exam and the exam will be the most accurate it can possibly be.

If you found this book helpful, please leave a review on Amazon, I would highly, highly appreciate it!

This will allow more people seeking natural ways to improve their eyesight a chance to come across it and the exercises, knowledge and information here can reach out to more people in need of it. In your review please don't hold back, tell me all the good and bad parts you liked about the book, I am always seeking feedback and wanting to improve in all endeavors of life.

Thank you and best of luck with your journey to 20/20 and beyond.

P.S. Don't forget your free bonus pack you can get on the next page!

CHAPTER 11 - FREE BONUSES

Guys, thank you so much for reading my book. I know it will serve you well on your journey as long as you TAKE ACTION and follow through with the 20/20 Vision Blueprint which is why I have compiled this nice little goodie bag for you guys to take with you on your journey.

There are four items in the bonus pack for you and I'll give a little run down with how each of them work.

1.   The 20/20 Vision Blueprint Excel Sheet + Instructions

This is an excel worksheet for you to print out and use to follow through on the 21-day program. Additional instructions can be found in the bonus pack as to how the program is structured with tips and suggestions for a successful 21 day program :)

2.   Eyesight Improvement: The 20/20 Vision Blueprint Book Summary

I am an avid reader and I love plowing through books but often find myself forgetting many of the points from great books so for your ease of use and comfort I have compiled the most noteworthy points from the book for you to refer to and glance at your leisure.

The best part about it is that all the E^2 Exercise instructions are included in it so that you can easily print them out and refer to them as you follow along with the program and not have to fiddle with your Kindle everytime.

3.   Tibetan Eye Chart

A Tibetan Eye Chart has been included for you to print off on an A4 sheet to be used with the Ancient Tibetan eye exercises outlined.

4.   Resource Cheat Sheet

The resource cheat sheet has links to my recommended products for the anglepoise lamp, pinhole glasses and links to eye chart tests with instructions on how to use them. The eye chart tests are all printable and easy to set up so you don't have to head to the optometrists each time to see how well you're progressing with the 20/20 Vision Blueprint. I have also provided links to a website I have contributed to in the past that provides A LOT of exercises on eyesight and instructions

Go to this link to claim your free bonus pack:

bit.ly/2020blueprint

As well as receiving the free bonus pack I will be in touch soon to check up on how you're doing with the program and will be more than glad to help with any questions you may have!

ABOUT THE AUTHOR

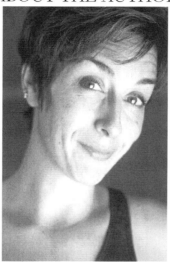

Joanne Bateman is a 32 year old entrepreneur who is a productivity and health freak. Prior to living the free life, her one and only full-time job she had was as a Store Manager for a large optometrist store chain in Michigan where she learned, used and developed natural eye exercises which she then started sharing with clients to improve their eyesight.

Surprisingly her reputation grew in the area and people started visiting her for private consultations and advice to naturally improve their eyesight. With suggestions from several of her clients to write a book and manual for what she taught *The 20/20 Vision Blueprint* eventually originated.

When she isn't spending time exploring, reading, doing yoga or Argentine Tango she can be found hunched over her laptop blogging, consulting with clients or spending time with her husband Jack and their lovely Siberian Husky Max.

INDEX

Printed in Great Britain
by Amazon.co.uk, Ltd.,
Marston Gate.